# UNVEILING AUTISM

## Exploring the Novel Aspects of Neurodiversity.

## By

## Sarah C. Ward

# TABLE OF CONTENTS

# Introduction

Unveiling Autism is a thought-provoking book that explores the complexities and challenges of living with autism, written by Sarah C. Ward, a mother, and advocate for individuals with autism. This book is an intimate portrayal of the author's journey, from the moment she learned of her son's diagnosis to the years of advocacy and dedication to helping others understand the disorder.

Sarah's journey with autism began when her son was just three years old. He had been experiencing difficulties with communication, social interaction, and sensory processing. After months of testing, Sarah and her husband were informed that their son had autism, a developmental disorder that affects an individual's ability to communicate, socialize, and behave appropriately.

At first, Sarah was devastated by the news. She was overwhelmed with questions and concerns about what the future would hold for her son. However, as she began to research autism, she realized that there was very little information available to parents like herself. She decided to take matters into her own hands and began studying the disorder and the best ways to support her son.

Over the years, Sarah's dedication to her son's development and progress led her to become an advocate for individuals with autism. She started attending conferences, networking with other parents and professionals, and learning everything she could about the disorder. She became a vocal advocate for autism awareness, speaking out about the importance of early intervention, education, and support.

As Sarah continued on her journey with autism, she discovered that there were many misconceptions and misunderstandings about the disorder. She realized that there was a need for a comprehensive guide to help parents, educators, and professionals better understand autism and how to support individuals on the spectrum. This led her to write Unveiling Autism, a detailed and insightful book that shares her personal experiences and provides practical advice and guidance to those impacted by the disorder.

Unveiling Autism is a unique book that offers an in-depth look at the challenges and triumphs of living with autism. Sarah's writing is engaging and insightful, and her personal stories provide a heartfelt and honest portrayal of the joys and struggles of raising a child with autism. Through her book, she aims to educate and inspire others, helping to break down the stigma and misconceptions that surround the disorder.

Throughout the pages of Unveiling Autism, readers will find a wealth of information and resources to help them better understand and support individuals with autism. Sarah covers topics such as early intervention, education, socialization, and communication, offering practical advice and real-world strategies for parents and professionals alike.
In addition to her personal experiences and insights, Sarah draws on the latest research and scientific findings in the field of autism to provide a comprehensive and up-to-date guide to the disorder. She also features interviews with other parents, professionals, and individuals with autism, offering a range of perspectives and experiences to help readers gain a deeper understanding of the disorder.

Unveiling Autism is a must-read for anyone impacted by autism, whether they are a parent, educator, or professional. Sarah's dedication to her son and her commitment to advocacy shine through on every page, making this book a powerful and inspiring resource for anyone seeking to better understand and support individuals with autism.

# Chapter One
# What Exactly is Autism?

Autism is a developmental disorder that affects a person's social communication and behavior. It is a spectrum disorder, which means that people with autism can have varying degrees of impairment. Some people with autism are highly functioning, while others require lifelong support and assistance. Autism is typically diagnosed in early childhood, and while there is no cure, early intervention, and therapy can help people with autism lead fulfilling lives.

As an author and a parent of a child with autism, I have spent years researching and learning about this complex disorder. In this chapter, I will provide an overview of what autism is, how it is diagnosed, and some of the common misconceptions about the disorder.

My son was diagnosed with autism when he was three years old. At the time, I knew very little about the disorder, and I was overwhelmed with fear and uncertainty about his future. But as I began to educate myself about autism, I learned that there is much more to this disorder than meets the eye.

Autism is a condition related to the development of the nervous system that impacts the manner in which an individual comprehends and interprets information.. People with autism may have difficulty with social communication and interaction, and they may engage in repetitive behaviors or have an intense interest in specific topics. Some people with autism may also have sensory sensitivities or challenges with motor coordination.

One of the most important things to understand about autism is that it is a spectrum disorder. This means that there is a wide range of abilities and challenges that people with autism can have. Some people with autism may have average or above-average intelligence, while others may have intellectual disabilities. Some may be able to live independently, while others may require lifelong support.

Autism is diagnosed through a comprehensive evaluation that includes observations of the person's behavior and communication, as well as interviews with the person and their family members. There is no single test that can diagnose autism, and it is important to have a thorough evaluation by a qualified professional.

One of the most common misconceptions about autism is that it is caused by bad parenting or social/environmental factors. This is not true. Autism is a neurodevelopmental disorder that is believed to have a genetic basis. While environmental factors may play a role in some cases, the cause of autism is not fully understood.

Another common misconception is that people with autism lack empathy or emotions. Again, this is not true. People with autism may have difficulty expressing their emotions or reading social cues, but they are capable of feeling emotions and forming strong connections with others.

In the following pages, I will share some real-life stories from my own experiences as a parent of a child with autism, as well as stories from other families who have been touched by this disorder. These stories will provide a glimpse into the challenges and triumphs of living with autism, and will hopefully help to dispel some of the myths and misconceptions about this disorder.

**Story 1: A Mother's Journey**

When my son was diagnosed with autism, I felt like my world had turned upside down. I had so many questions and fears about his future. Would he be able to make friends? Would he be able to live independently? Would he be able to communicate his thoughts and feelings? I was overwhelmed with uncertainty.

But as I began to educate myself about autism, I realized that my son was not defined by his diagnosis. He was still the same amazing, curious, and loving child that he had always been. His perspective of the world was unique.

Through early intervention and therapy, my son has made incredible progress. He has learned to communicate his thoughts and feelings, and he has developed a love for music and art. He still faces challenges, but he has also shown incredible resilience and determination.

My journey as a mother of a child with autism has been filled with both heartache and joy. But it has also taught me so much about compassion, acceptance, and the power of love. I have learned to celebrate my son's strengths and to support him in his challenges.

I have also had the privilege of connecting with other families who have children with autism. Through support groups and online communities, I have found a network of people who understand the unique challenges and joys of raising a child with autism. These connections have been a source of strength and encouragement for me on my journey.

**Story 2: A Family's Triumph**

When James was diagnosed with autism at the age of five, his parents were devastated. They had always known that he was different, but they had never imagined that their son would have a lifelong disorder.

But as they began to learn more about autism, James's parents realized that their son was not defined by his diagnosis. He was still the same creative and loving child that he had always been. They decided to focus on his strengths and support him in his challenges.

Through therapy and early intervention, James made incredible progress. He developed a love for music and art, and he began to communicate his thoughts and feelings more effectively. He also developed a strong interest in science and technology, and his parents supported this interest by enrolling him in coding classes and science camps.

Today, James is a successful software engineer and a passionate advocate for people with autism. He uses his own experiences to raise awareness and inspire others to embrace their differences and pursue their passions.

These stories are just a few examples of the many families who have been touched by autism. While autism can be a challenging disorder, it is also a disorder that can bring out the best in people. People with autism often have unique talents and perspectives, and they can make significant contributions to society.

In the following chapters, we will delve deeper into the challenges and opportunities of living with autism. We will explore the various therapies and interventions that can help people with autism thrive, and we will discuss the importance of early intervention and support.

We will also explore the impact of autism on families and caregivers, and we will provide practical tips and strategies for navigating the challenges of daily life. Our hope is that this book will serve as a valuable resource for families and caregivers who are navigating the complex and often overwhelming world of autism.

# Chapter Two
# Who are the Veiled Autistics?

In recent years, the term "veiling" has gained significant attention in the autism community. Veiling refers to the practice of concealing one's autistic traits in order to fit in with neurotypical society. Veiling can manifest in various ways, including social mimicry, imitation of others' behaviors, and suppression of autistic stims.

Many autistic individuals report that veiling comes at a significant cost to their mental health, as it requires constant vigilance and effort to maintain. Despite this, masking is often necessary for autistic individuals to navigate a world that is not designed with their needs in mind.

In this chapter, we will explore the concept of masking in greater depth, including its prevalence, impact, and potential benefits and drawbacks. We will also hear from autistic individuals who have experience with veiling, including the author's own personal stories.

## Prevalence of Veiling

Veiling is a common experience among autistic individuals, especially those who were not diagnosed until later in life. In fact, research suggests that many autistic individuals engage in some form of veiling behavior to varying degrees.

A study conducted by the Autism Research Centre found that individuals who were diagnosed with autism later in life were more likely to report veiling than those who were diagnosed earlier. This suggests that early diagnosis and intervention may help reduce the need for masking and improve autistic individuals' overall well-being.

However, even among those who are diagnosed early, veiling may still be necessary for certain situations. For example, autistic individuals may feel pressure to mask their autistic traits in order to fit in with their neurotypical peers at school or work.

## Impact of Veiling

Veiling can have a significant impact on an autistic individual's mental health and well-being. Many autistic individuals report feeling exhausted and burned out from constantly suppressing their natural behaviors and instincts.

In addition, veiling can lead to a sense of disconnection from one's true self, as the individual is constantly performing a role in order to fit in with others. This can lead to feelings of anxiety, depression, and social isolation.

One study found that autistic individuals who engaged in more masking behaviors also reported higher levels of anxiety and depression. This suggests that masking may be a contributing factor to poor mental health outcomes for autistic individuals.

## Benefits and Drawbacks of Veiling

While veiling can be exhausting and detrimental to mental health, some autistic individuals may feel that it is necessary in order to navigate certain situations. For example, autistic individuals may feel that they need to mask their stimming behaviors in order to avoid negative attention from others.

In some cases, veiling may also provide certain benefits. For example, an autistic individual may be able to pass as neurotypical in certain situations, which can help them avoid discrimination and gain access to resources and opportunities that may be otherwise unavailable to them.

However, these benefits must be weighed against the potential costs of masking. For many autistic individuals, the toll of veiling can be significant and may outweigh any perceived benefits.

**Personal Stories**
As an autistic individual, the author has firsthand experience with veiling. Throughout her life, the author has felt pressure to veil her autistic traits in order to fit in with her neurotypical peers.

For example, in elementary school, the author learned to mimic her classmates' behaviors in order to avoid standing out. She would watch what other children did and try to copy them, even if it felt unnatural or uncomfortable.

In high school, the author felt pressure to hide her stimming behaviors, such as rocking and hand-flapping, in order to avoid being teased or bullied by their classmates. This required a great deal of effort and self-control, and often left the author feeling exhausted and disconnected from their true self.

As an adult, the author has continued to mask in certain situations, such as job interviews or social gatherings where she feels that her autistic traits may be stigmatized or misunderstood. However, the author has also learned to embrace her autistic identity and prioritize her own well-being over the pressure to conform to societal expectations.

The author has also spoken with other autistic individuals who have experienced masking in various ways. One individual, who was not diagnosed with autism until adulthood, described feeling like he had spent his entire life pretending to be someone he was not. He recounted numerous instances where he had suppressed his natural behaviors in order to fit in with neurotypical society and expressed a sense of sadness and frustration at the toll this had taken on his mental health.

Another individual described feeling like she was constantly performing a role in order to fit in with others. She explained that she had learned to mimic the behaviors and mannerisms of their neurotypical peers in order to avoid standing out, but that this had come at a significant cost to her sense of self.

In conclusion, masking is a common experience among autistic individuals and can have a significant impact on their mental health and well-being. While veiling may be necessary for certain situations, such as to avoid discrimination or gain access to resources and opportunities, it is important to acknowledge the potential costs of this practice.

As a society, we must work to create more inclusive and accepting environments for autistic individuals, where they can feel safe to express their true selves without fear of stigma or discrimination. This requires a shift in attitudes and perceptions around autism, and a recognition of the valuable contributions that autistic individuals can make to our communities. By listening to and learning from the experiences of autistic individuals, we can work towards a more equitable and just society for all.

# Chapter Three
# The Structure and Components of the Veil

Autism is often referred to as the "invisible disability" due to the hidden nature of its symptoms. Individuals with autism may have difficulty with social interactions, communication, and sensory processing, but these challenges are not always immediately apparent to others. As a result, many individuals with autism develop coping mechanisms to navigate the social world, often referred to as "veiling"

In this chapter, we will explore the structure and components of the veil, by examining the different ways in which individuals with autism may veil their symptoms and the impact that veiling can have on their well-being.

## What is Veiling?

Veiling refers to the process of hiding or suppressing one's autistic traits or behaviors in order to fit in or conform to social expectations. Veiling can take many different forms, from mimicking social behaviors that do not come naturally to an individual with autism to suppressing stimming behaviors or special interests.

Veiling can be a useful coping mechanism for individuals with autism, allowing them to navigate social situations more easily and avoid negative reactions from others. However, masking can also be incredibly stressful and exhausting, leading to burnout and mental health issues over time.

**Types of Veiling**
There are many different ways in which individuals with autism may mask their symptoms. Here are a few examples:

**1 Mimicking Social Behaviors**
Individuals with autism may learn to mimic social behaviors that do not come naturally to them, such as making eye contact, maintaining appropriate personal space, or engaging in small talk. While this can help them blend in, it can also be incredibly stressful and exhausting.

## 2 Suppressing Stimming Behaviors

Stimming behaviors are repetitive movements or sounds that individuals with autism may engage in as a way of self-soothing or regulating their sensory input. These behaviors can include hand flapping, rocking back and forth, or repeating certain phrases. In order to avoid negative reactions from others, individuals with autism may learn to suppress these behaviors, which can lead to increased anxiety and stress.

## 3 Veiling Special Interests

Special interests are intense and passionate interests that individuals with autism may develop in specific topics or activities. While these interests can be a source of joy and fulfillment, they can also be socially stigmatized. In order to avoid negative reactions from others, individuals with autism may learn to mask or hide their special interests.

## The Impact of Veiling

While veiling can be a useful coping mechanism in the short term, it can have a significant impact on the well-being of individuals with autism in the long term. Here are a few examples:

## 1 Burnout

Masking requires a great deal of mental and emotional energy, which can lead to burnout over time. Individuals with autism who engage in masking may experience exhaustion, anxiety, and depression as a result.

## 2 Identity Issues

Veiling can also lead to confusion about one's identity. Individuals with autism who mask their symptoms may feel like they are living a double life, with one persona for the public world and one for their private self.

## 3 Social Isolation

Veiling can make it difficult for individuals with autism to connect with others on a deeper level. If they are not able to express their true selves, they may struggle to form meaningful relationships or find acceptance and understanding.

**Supporting Individuals with Autism**

In order to support individuals with autism, it is important to recognize the impact of masking and provide them with the tools and resources they need to be themselves. Below are some approaches that may prove beneficial.

**1 Create Safe Spaces**

Provide individuals with autism with safe spaces where they can be themselves without fear of judgment or negative reactions.

**2 Normalize Differences**

Encourage others to embrace and celebrate differences rather than conform to a narrow definition of "normal."

**3 Educate Others**

Educate friends, family members, and others about autism and the challenges that individuals with autism face. By increasing awareness and understanding, we can help to create a more inclusive and accepting society.

**4 Advocate for Accommodations**

Individuals with autism may benefit from accommodations in school, work, and other settings. Advocate for these accommodations to be provided and ensure that they are accessible and effective.

**5 Support Self-Expression**

Encourage individuals with autism to express themselves in ways that feel comfortable and natural to them. This may mean allowing them to stimulate or pursue their special interests without judgment or criticism.

By taking these steps, we can help to create a more accepting and supportive environment for individuals with autism. Instead of masking their symptoms and struggling to fit in, they can feel confident and empowered to be themselves. In doing so, we can all benefit from the unique perspectives and talents that individuals with autism bring to the world.

# Chapter Four
# The Price of Veiling

The topic of veiling has received increasing attention in the autism community in recent years. Veiling refers to the practice of hiding one's autistic traits and behaviors in order to fit in with neurotypical society. Masking can take many forms, from suppressing stimming behaviors to forcing oneself to make eye contact. While masking can help individuals with autism navigate social situations more easily, it can also have serious long-term consequences.

In this chapter, we will explore the price of veiling for individuals with autism. We will discuss the physical, emotional, and psychological toll that veiling can take, as well as the impact on social and communication skills. We will also explore strategies for reducing the need to mask and promoting self-acceptance.

## The Physical Cost of Veiling

Veiling can have a number of physical consequences. One of the most common is fatigue. Many individuals with autism report feeling exhausted after social interactions or other situations where they feel they must mask their true selves. This can lead to a cycle of avoidance, where individuals with autism may withdraw from social situations in order to conserve energy.

Another physical consequence of masking is increased stress levels. When individuals with autism feel they must constantly suppress their natural behaviors, they can experience a range of physical symptoms, from headaches to stomachaches. This chronic stress can also weaken the immune system, making individuals more susceptible to illness.

## The Emotional Cost of Veiling

Veiling can also take a significant emotional toll. Many individuals with autism report feeling like they are living a double life, constantly hiding their true selves from the world. Such circumstances can result in emotions of seclusion, solitude, and possibly melancholy.

Furthermore, masking can erode self-esteem. When individuals with autism feel they must hide who they are in order to be accepted, they may begin to internalize negative messages about themselves. Such a situation may result in an unfavorable perception of oneself and insufficient belief in one's abilities.

**The Psychological Cost of Veiling**
Veiling can also have serious psychological consequences. Many individuals with autism report feeling like they have lost a sense of themselves, as they spend so much time trying to fit in with neurotypical society. A variety of mental health problems, such as anxiety and depression, may arise as a result of this.

Furthermore, masking can hinder the development of social and communication skills. When individuals with autism are constantly suppressing their natural behaviors, they may miss out on opportunities to learn and practice social skills. This can make it even harder for them to navigate social situations in the future.

**Reducing the Need to Veil:**

While it may not be possible to completely eliminate the need to veil, there are strategies that individuals with autism can use to reduce the amount of masking they must do. These strategies include:

1 Finding safe spaces where individuals can be themselves without fear of judgment or ridicule.

2 Building a support network of individuals who understand and accept them for who they are.

3 Practicing self-care, including exercise, meditation, and other stress-reducing activities.

4 Seeking therapy or counseling to work through issues related to masking and self-acceptance.

## Promoting Self-Acceptance

Ultimately, the key to reducing the negative effects of masking is promoting self-acceptance. When individuals with autism are able to embrace and celebrate their unique traits and behaviors, they are less likely to feel the need to mask. This can lead to increased self-confidence, improved social and communication skills, and better overall mental health.

In conclusion, masking can have serious consequences for individuals with autism, both physically and emotionally. However, by reducing the need to mask and promoting self-acceptance, individuals with autism can learn to thrive in a world that may not always understand them

# Chapter Five
# Reevaluating the Concept of Autism

Autism has been a topic of discussion for decades, with different theories and perspectives on what it is and how it should be treated. However, as more research is done and more people with autism share their experiences, it is becoming clear that the traditional understanding of autism needs to be rethought.

In this chapter, we will explore the current understanding of autism, the limitations of this understanding, and new ways of thinking about autism that have the potential to improve the lives of people with autism.

## Autism: A Spectrum of Differences

Autism is a condition that impacts the development of the nervous system and can lead to difficulties in communication, social interaction, and behavior. It is typically diagnosed in early childhood, and the severity of symptoms can vary widely from person to person.

The traditional view of autism is that it is a set of deficits or impairments. People with autism are often described as lacking social skills, being unable to read social cues, and having difficulty with communication. They may also engage in repetitive behaviors or have narrow interests.

However, this view of autism is limited in several ways. First, it focuses on what people with autism cannot do, rather than what they can do. People with autism may have unique strengths and abilities, such as a strong memory or an intense focus on a particular subject.

Secondly, the traditional view of autism does not account for the wide range of experiences that people with autism have. Autism is a spectrum disorder, which means that there is a broad range of symptoms and severity levels. Some people with autism may have very few symptoms and be able to function well in society, while others may require significant support to navigate everyday life.

Finally, the traditional view of autism assumes that the goal of treatment is to make people with autism more "normal." This assumes that there is a single, correct way to be and that people with autism need to be fixed in order to fit into this mold. However, this view ignores the fact that people with autism have unique experiences and perspectives that should be valued and celebrated.

## A New Understanding of Autism

In recent years, there has been a growing recognition that the traditional view of autism is limiting and incomplete. Instead, a new understanding of autism is emerging, one that recognizes the diversity of experiences and the unique strengths and abilities of people with autism.

This new understanding of autism is often referred to as the neurodiversity movement. The neurodiversity movement asserts that autism is not a disorder or a deficit, but a natural variation in the human brain. People with autism are not broken or in need of fixing; they are simply different.

The neurodiversity movement argues that people with autism should be accepted and celebrated for who they are, rather than being forced to conform to neurotypical standards. This means creating environments that are inclusive and accommodating to people with autism, rather than trying to make them fit into environments that are designed for neurotypical people.

The neurodiversity movement also recognizes that people with autism have unique strengths and abilities. For example, many people with autism have excellent attention to detail, strong problem-solving skills, and a deep understanding of certain subjects. These strengths can be valuable in many different fields and should be recognized and encouraged.

**Implications for Treatment**

The shift towards a neurodiversity perspective has important implications for how autism is treated. Instead of focusing on fixing deficits, the goal of treatment should be to support people with autism in achieving their goals and reaching their full potential.

This means providing accommodations and support to help people with autism navigate the challenges of everyday life. For example, providing sensory-friendly environments, offering communication devices or apps, and allowing for flexible schedules can all help people with autism thrive.

It also means valuing and encouraging the unique strengths and abilities of people with autism. This may involve providing opportunities for people with autism to pursue their interests and passions, rather than trying to force them to conform to traditional expectations. For example, a person with autism who has a deep interest in mathematics could be encouraged to pursue a career in a maths-related field, rather than being pushed toward a more "typical" career path.

Another important aspect of treatment is providing support for mental health and well-being. People with autism are at increased risk for conditions such as anxiety and depression and may struggle with feelings of isolation or social rejection. By providing support and resources to address these challenges, we can help people with autism lead happier and more fulfilling lives.

**The Importance of Listening to People with Autism**

As we rethink our understanding of autism and the best ways to support people with autism, it is essential that we listen to the perspectives and experiences of people with autism themselves. Far too often, the voices of people with autism have been ignored or dismissed in discussions about their own lives and experiences.

One way to ensure that people with autism are heard is by involving them in research and advocacy efforts. By working together with people with autism, researchers and advocates can gain a deeper understanding of the challenges and strengths associated with autism, and develop more effective strategies for supporting people with autism.

Another way to listen to people with autism is by creating spaces for them to share their own stories and perspectives. This could involve creating support groups, hosting community events, or providing online platforms for people with autism to connect and share their experiences.

In this chapter, we have explored the traditional view of autism as a set of deficits or impairments, and the limitations of this understanding. We have also discussed the emerging neurodiversity perspective, which recognizes autism as a natural variation in the human brain and values the unique strengths and abilities of people with autism.

As we continue to rethink our understanding of autism and the best ways to support people with autism, it is essential that we listen to the perspectives and experiences of people with autism themselves. By working together with people with autism, we can create a more inclusive and accommodating society that values and celebrates the diversity of human experiences

# Chapter Six
# Developing Relationships with Autistic Individuals

Autism is a complex neurological condition that affects communication, social interaction, and behavior. As a result, individuals with autism may have difficulty building and maintaining relationships. Cultivating autistic relationships requires patience, understanding, and a willingness to learn about autism.

In this chapter, we will explore strategies for cultivating autistic relationships. We will also hear from individuals with autism and their families about their experiences with building and maintaining relationships.

**Understanding Autism**

Before we dive into strategies for cultivating autistic relationships, it's important to have a basic understanding of autism. Autism is a spectrum condition, which means that it affects individuals in different ways and to varying degrees. However, there are some common characteristics of autism, including

## 1 Difficulty with social communication and interaction

Individuals with autism may struggle with social communication, such as understanding nonverbal cues, taking turns in conversation, and interpreting sarcasm or jokes. They may also have difficulty with social interaction, such as making friends and understanding social rules.

## 2 Restricted and repetitive behaviors and interests

Restricted and repetitive behaviors and interests can include a narrow focus on one particular topic or activity, repetitive behaviors such as hand-flapping or rocking, and a need for routine and predictability.

## 3 Sensory sensitivities

Sensory sensitivities can manifest in a variety of ways, such as being sensitive to certain textures, sounds, or smells.

It's important to keep in mind that each individual with autism is unique, and may experience these characteristics in different ways. Understanding and accepting these differences is key to cultivating autistic relationships.

**Strategies for Cultivating Autistic Relationships**
Now that we have a basic understanding of autism, let's explore some strategies for cultivating autistic relationships.

**1 Be Patient**
Individuals with autism may need more time to process information and respond to social cues. It's important to be patient and allow them the time they need to communicate in their own way. This can include using visual supports, such as pictures or social stories, to help them understand social situations.

**2 Use Clear and Direct Language:**
Individuals with autism may have difficulty understanding figurative language, sarcasm, or jokes. When interacting with them, it's crucial to employ straightforward and unambiguous language. This can include avoiding idioms and metaphors and being specific about what you mean.

**3 Be Understanding**

Individuals with autism may have difficulty with sensory sensitivities or may become overwhelmed in social situations. It's important to be understanding and provide support when needed. This can include offering a quiet space to retreat to or providing noise-canceling headphones.

**4 Focus on Shared Interests**

Individuals with autism may have a narrow focus on one particular topic or activity. Focusing on shared interests can be a great way to build a connection and cultivate a relationship. This can include engaging in a favorite activity together or discussing a shared interest.

**5 Embrace Differences**

Individuals with autism may have different ways of communicating or interacting socially. It's important to embrace these differences and not try to force them to conform to neurotypical social norms. This can include accepting stimming behaviors or allowing for more time to process information.

## Real-Life Experiences

Now, let's hear from individuals with autism and their families about their experiences with building and maintaining relationships.

## Lucas's Story

Lucas is a 12-year-old boy with autism. He loves trains and can recite every train schedule in the country. Lucas has difficulty with social communication and interaction and often struggles to make friends.

Lucas's mother, Maria, has found that focusing on Lucas's interests has helped them build a stronger relationship. They often visit train museums together and discuss the different types of trains. Maria also uses social stories to help Lucas understand social situations."Lucas is such a wonderful boy, and I feel grateful every day that he is my son," Maria said. "Building a relationship with him has had its challenges, but focusing on his interests and communicating in a way that he can understand has made all the difference. Lucas has taught me so much about patience, empathy, and acceptance."

Maria also emphasized the importance of seeking support from professionals and other families who have experience with autism.She stated that although it can feel daunting and lonely at times, discovering a supportive community has been extremely valuable.

**Mark's Story**
Mark is a 25-year-old man with autism. He has a passion for music and can play the guitar and piano with exceptional skill. Mark has struggled with social communication and has found it challenging to make friends.

Mark's father, John, has been a strong advocate for his son and has supported him in pursuing his musical interests. John has helped Mark find opportunities to perform and has connected him with other musicians who share his passion.

John expressed his pride in Mark, stating that he possesses a truly exceptional talent. "Building a relationship with him has been a journey, but I've learned to accept and embrace his differences. It's

important to focus on his strengths and provide opportunities for him to pursue his passions."
John also stressed the importance of finding the right support and services for individuals with autism. He stated that although it may seem like a daunting task to navigate the system, locating suitable professionals and programs can have a significant impact

In conclusion, cultivating autistic relationships requires patience, understanding, and a willingness to learn about autism. By focusing on shared interests, using clear and direct language, and embracing differences, we can build strong and meaningful relationships with individuals with autism.

As we have heard from Lucas and Mark's stories, supporting individuals with autism in pursuing their passions and finding the right support and services can also make a significant impact. By working together, we can create a world where individuals with autism are accepted, valued, and celebrated for who they are.

# Chapter Seven
# Building a World that Embraces Neurodiversity

In this chapter, we explore the concept of neurodiversity and how it can lead to a more inclusive and accepting world. We will discuss the importance of accommodating different ways of thinking and learning, and how this can benefit not only those with neurodivergent traits but society as a whole.

Neurodiversity is the idea that neurological differences, such as autism, ADHD, dyslexia, and others, are not disorders or deficits but variations of human experience. Instead of trying to cure or fix these differences, we should embrace them and create an environment that allows everyone to thrive. This includes providing accommodations, support, and acceptance for individuals with neurodivergent traits.

As someone who identifies as autistic, I have experienced first-hand the challenges and discrimination that can arise from being neurodivergent. But I have also seen the beauty and strengths that can come from embracing neurodiversity. In this chapter, I will share some of my personal experiences and those of others in the autistic community to illustrate the importance of creating a neurodiverse world.

**Embracing Neurodiversity**

When we think of diversity, we often think of differences in race, gender, and culture. However, neurodiversity is an equally important aspect of diversity that is often overlooked. We can foster a more inclusive and accepting society by accepting and valuing the diversity of neurological differences.

One way to embrace neurodiversity is by providing accommodations for individuals with neurodivergent traits. These accommodations can include things like sensory-friendly environments, alternative communication methods, and flexible work schedules. By providing these accommodations, we can create a more accessible world for everyone.

Another way to embrace neurodiversity is by recognizing and valuing the strengths that come with neurodivergent traits. For example, individuals with autism may have exceptional attention to detail or a unique way of problem-solving. By recognizing and valuing these strengths, we can create a more diverse and productive workforce.

**Overcoming Barriers**

Despite the benefits of neurodiversity, there are still many barriers that prevent individuals with neurodivergent traits from fully participating in society. These barriers can include stigma, discrimination, and lack of understanding.

One of the biggest barriers for individuals with neurodivergent traits is the lack of understanding and awareness about these conditions. Many people still view autism and other neurodivergent traits as disorders or deficits, rather than variations of human experience. This can lead to stereotypes and discrimination, which can further marginalize individuals with these traits.

Another barrier for individuals with neurodivergent traits is the lack of accommodations and support. Without these accommodations, individuals with neurodivergent traits may struggle to navigate everyday life, including school, work, and social situations. This can lead to isolation and exclusion from society.

**Personal Stories**
In this section, I will share some personal stories from myself and others in the autistic community. These stories illustrate the challenges and triumphs of being neurodivergent and highlight the importance of creating a neurodiverse world.

**Story One: My Journey to Self-Acceptance**
For many years, I struggled to accept my autism. I felt like an outsider and often tried to mask my differences in order to fit in. It wasn't until I found a supportive community of other autistic individuals that I began to embrace my neurodivergent traits. Through this community, I learned that being different is not a bad thing and that my autism is a part of who I am. Today, I am proud to be autistic and advocate for neurodiversity.

**Story Two: The Importance of Accommodations**
John is a young man with autism who struggled in school due to sensory overload and difficulty with social interactions. Despite his challenges, John was determined to succeed and worked hard to develop coping strategies and accommodations that would help him navigate the school environment. With the help of a supportive teacher, John was able to create a sensory-friendly workspace and schedule that allowed him to focus on his studies without being overwhelmed by sensory input. He also received social skills training and was able to develop friendships with his peers. Today, John is a successful college graduate and advocates for the importance of accommodations and support for individuals with neurodivergent traits.

**Story Three: Overcoming Stereotypes**

Samantha is a young woman with autism who was often underestimated and dismissed because of her differences. People would assume that she was unable to communicate or understand complex concepts, simply because of her autism. However, Samantha was determined to prove them wrong. She developed a love for coding and programming and worked hard to develop her skills. Through her work, Samantha was able to show that autism does not define her abilities or potential. Today, Samantha is a successful software engineer and advocates for the importance of recognizing and valuing the strengths of neurodivergent individuals.

**Creating a Neurodiverse World**

In order to create a neurodiverse world, we must work together to overcome the barriers and challenges that prevent individuals with neurodivergent traits from fully participating in society. This includes:

1 Educating ourselves and others about neurodiversity and the strengths and challenges that come with neurodivergent traits.

2 Providing accommodations and support for individuals with neurodivergent traits in all areas of life, including school, work, and social situations.

3 Recognizing and valuing the strengths of neurodivergent individuals and creating a more diverse and inclusive workforce.

4 Challenging stereotypes and discrimination that perpetuate stigma and exclusion.

By working together to create a neurodiverse world, we can create a more inclusive and accepting society that benefits everyone. It is my hope that this chapter has inspired you to embrace neurodiversity and advocate for the rights and needs of individuals with neurodivergent traits.

# Conclusion

In conclusion, Unveiling Autism is a deeply personal and insightful book that sheds light on the complexities and challenges of living with autism. Written by Sarah, a mother and advocate for individuals with autism, this book offers a wealth of knowledge, resources, and practical advice to help parents, educators, and professionals better understand and support those on the spectrum.

Throughout the book, Sarah shares her personal journey with autism, from the moment she learned of her son's diagnosis to her years of advocacy and dedication to helping others. Her writing is engaging and heartfelt, offering an honest portrayal of the joys and struggles of raising a child with autism. Through her stories and experiences, readers gain a deeper understanding of the impact of autism on individuals and their families.

One of the key themes of Unveiling Autism is the importance of early intervention and support. Sarah emphasizes the need for parents and professionals to work together to identify and address the unique needs of each individual on the spectrum. She provides practical advice and real-world strategies for supporting individuals with autism in areas such as education, socialization, and communication.

Another important theme of the book is the need to break down the stigma and misconceptions that surround autism. Sarah highlights the importance of autism awareness and acceptance and encourages readers to become advocates for individuals with autism. Through her advocacy work, she hopes to change the way that society views and treats those on the spectrum.

One of the strengths of Unveiling Autism is the comprehensive and up-to-date information that Sarah provides. She draws on the latest research and scientific findings in the field of autism to offer a comprehensive guide to the disorder. She also features interviews with other parents, professionals, and individuals with autism, offering a range of perspectives and experiences to help readers gain a deeper understanding of the disorder.

Overall, Unveiling Autism is a powerful and inspiring book that offers hope and guidance to anyone impacted by autism. Sarah's dedication to her son and her commitment to advocacy shine through on every page, making this book a valuable resource for anyone seeking to better understand and support individuals with autism. By sharing her personal journey and insights, she has created a book that will resonate with readers and inspire them to make a difference in the lives of those on the spectrum.